The Business of Fitness Supplements

Creating and Selling Nutritional Products

Introduction

The world continues its search for the secret alchemy to optimal health, vitality, and fitness. More than ever, fitness supplements are at the core of this quest. People are harnessing the power of nutritional supplements to maximise their fitness levels and improve their overall health. This has evolved into a booming industry across the globe.

"The Business of Fitness Supplements: Creating and Selling Nutritional Products" is a comprehensive exploration into this explosive industry. The allure and potential profitability of the supplement sector have beckoned many entrepreneurs and corporations, but what does it truly take to create a successful brand in this busy marketplace? This book aims to answer that question and many more.

It begins by demystifying the science and categories of fitness supplements, taking readers through the essential constituents and their respective roles in enhancing fitness. We then delve into the dynamics of the global supplement market, discussing the dominant players, key trends, and considerable market shifts.

The heart of this book will unravel the process of creating a fitness supplement, from imagining the initial product to taking it into full-scale production. Essential considerations such as branding, packaging, marketing, and selling strategies are discussed at length, with practical insights and proven tactics.

Consumer behaviour and its influence on the purchasing process forms another integral aspect of our discussion, helping to unveil the secrets of connecting with the target market and driving sales. Furthermore, we underline the importance of staying compliant in this highly regulated industry, outlining some common legal pitfalls and how best to avoid them.

Lastly, we take a glimpse beyond the horizon at the future direction of fitness supplements, highlighting upcoming trends and potential areas of growth. As a whole, the reading journey promises to offer invaluable insights for aspiring entrepreneurs, seasoned professionals, or even fitness enthusiasts curious about the supplements they consume.

Welcome to "The Business of Fitness Supplements: Creating and Selling Nutritional Products", where we unravel the complexities, challenges, and opportunities of one of the most dynamic and lucrative industries on the planet. Join us as we chart a course through the dense, vibrant jungle of the supplement industry, where science, business, regulation, and innovation intertwine.

Chapter one
Introduction to Fitness Supplements

1.1 Importance of Fitness Supplements in Modern Lifestyle

In an age where modern living often means increased sedentaryism, higher stress levels, and less-than-optimal eating habits, fitness supplements have emerged as an essential component of daily life for millions of people worldwide. These supplements serve as supportive measures designed to bridge nutritional gaps, enabling us to achieve our fitness, wellness, and performance goals. In this chapter, we will explore the importance of fitness supplements in the modern lifestyle and how they have become a crucial part of our daily routines.

1 Compensating for Nutritional Deficiencies

Due to the fast pace of modern life, our diets frequently fall short in providing all the necessary nutrients for optimal health. Consuming processed and convenience foods, while time-saving, often results in inadequate micronutrient intake and higher levels of unhealthy fats and sugars. Fitness supplements help make up for these deficiencies and keep our bodies functioning properly. They can offer essential vitamins, minerals, and nutrients to support our immune systems, maintain balanced energy levels, and promote muscle growth and recovery.

2 Enhancing Athletic Performance

For athletes and fitness enthusiasts, sport-specific supplements offer an extra edge, helping improve performance, speed up recovery, and increase stamina. Popular supplements such as protein powders for muscle growth, pre-workout formulas to enhance focus, and electrolyte supplements for hydration play a vital role in achieving peak athletic performance. Advanced supplement ingredients like branched-chain amino acids (BCAAs) and creatine have become indispensable tools for many athletes and bodybuilders.

3 Managing Stress and Boosting Energy Levels

Modern life demands long hours of work, disrupted sleeping patterns, and chronic stress, leading to a widespread need for supplements that minimize the impact of these factors on our overall well-being. Adaptogenic herbs and supplements like ashwagandha, rhodiola, and ginseng have become popular for their stress-relieving properties. Nootropic supplements, designed to enhance memory, focus, and cognitive function, have also garnered attention as people search for ways to maximize productivity and mental capacity.

4 Supporting Weight Loss and Body Composition

With obesity on the rise globally, people are increasingly turning to supplements to help manage their weight and reach their fitness goals. Fat burners, thermogenic stimulants, and appetite suppressants provide varying levels of support in conjunction with healthy eating plans and regular exercise. Moreover, high-quality fitness supplements like whey protein isolate and vegan protein powders that aid in weight loss and muscle gain are becoming staples in many weight management regimens.

5 Enhancing Overall Health and Well-being

In addition to their specific fitness-related benefits, many supplements help maintain general health and well-being by providing antioxidants, anti-inflammatory compounds, and immune support. Supplements like omega-3 fatty acids, multivitamins, green superfood blends, and probiotics provide essential nutrients and support for a healthy lifestyle, allowing us to operate in top form on a daily basis. These supplements also contribute to the prevention and alleviation of certain health conditions in conjunction with proper medical guidance.

Chapter two

Understanding Fitness Supplements

2.1 Categories of Fitness Supplements

As we deepen our understanding of fitness supplements and their significance in the modern world, it's essential to examine the various categories within this industry and the unique benefits each type offers. There are numerous kinds of fitness supplements, each designed to address specific aspects of health, fitness, and well-being, catering to a wide range of consumer needs. In this section, we explore the main categories of fitness supplements, providing a comprehensive overview that will enable readers to make informed decisions in the realm of supplementation.

1 Protein Powders

Protein powders serve as a primary source of dietary protein supplementation. They promote muscle growth, repair, and recovery, making them immensely popular among athletes, bodybuilders, and fitness enthusiasts. The most common types of protein powders include:

- Whey Protein

- Casein Protein

- Vegan Proteins (Soy, Pea, Rice, Hemp)

2 Amino Acids and BCAAs

Amino acids are the building blocks of proteins and serve as the foundation for muscle tissue growth. Branched-Chain Amino Acids (BCAAs), comprising leucine, isoleucine, and valine, are particularly important for enhancing muscle recovery and reducing muscle soreness.

3 Creatine

Creatine is a natural compound found in meat and fish that aids in the production of adenosine triphosphate (ATP), which powers our muscles during high-intensity exercise. Creatine supplements have been proven effective in enhancing muscle strength, power, and overall performance.

4 Pre-Workout Formulas

Pre-workout supplements are designed to provide energy, focus, and endurance during intense training sessions. They usually contain a combination of stimulants like caffeine, amino acids, vitamins, and minerals, among other ingredients, to optimize athletic performance.

5 Fat Burners and Thermogenics

These supplements support weight loss goals by increasing metabolism, suppressing appetite, and enhancing the body's fat-burning capabilities. Ingredients like green tea extract, caffeine, and capsaicin (found in hot peppers) are common components of fat burners.

6 Vitamins and Minerals

Vitamins and minerals are vital mioronutrients that support various bodily processes. Multivitamin supplements contain a balanced blend of essential vitamins and minerals to fill in dietary gaps and promote overall health.

7 Omega-3 Fatty Acids

Omega-3 fatty acids, namely EPA and DHA, are essential nutrients that support brain function, cognitive health, cardiovascular health, and reduce inflammation in our bodies. Fish oil, krill oil, and plant-based sources like algae are popular omega-3 supplements.

8 Probiotics and Digestive Enzymes

Probiotics consist of beneficial bacteria that help maintain gut health, digestion, and enhance immune function. Digestive enzyme supplements, on the other hand, break down food molecules to aid in digestion and nutrient absorption.

9 Joint Support

Joint support supplements typically contain a mix of ingredients that promote joint health, alleviate joint pain, and reduce inflammation. Common ingredients include glucosamine, chondroitin, MSM (methylsulfonylmethane), and hyaluronic acid.

10 Testosterone Boosters and Hormone Support

Designed to optimize hormonal balance, testosterone boosters and hormone support supplements are popular among male athletes and older men seeking increased strength, stamina, and improved sexual performance. These supplements often contain natural ingredients like D-aspartic acid, fenugreek, and Tribulus terrestris.

2.2 Importance and Role of Each Supplement

To fully appreciate the benefits of fitness supplements in the pursuit of health and wellness, it's essential to recognize the distinct roles and importance of each supplement type. This knowledge will enable consumers to make tailored decisions and develop an optimized supplementation plan to support their goals and respond to their bodies' unique needs. In this section, we shed light on the crucial roles and significance of each type of fitness supplement, empowering individuals to make informed choices.

1 Protein Powders

The role of protein powders in muscle building, repair, and recovery cannot be understated. They provide a convenient and easily digestible source of high-quality protein required for optimum muscle growth, preventing muscle breakdown (catabolism), and aiding in post-workout recovery. Protein powders are an essential addition to the supplement regimen of athletes, bodybuilders, and individuals looking to maintain or increase their lean muscle mass.

2 Amino Acids and BCAAs

Amino acids play critical roles in signalling, enzyme function, and neurotransmitter production in the body.

BCAAs, specifically, are essential for promoting muscle protein synthesis, sparing muscle glycogen, reducing muscle breakdown, and accelerating recovery. BCAAs also offer potential benefits in attenuating exercise-induced fatigue and boosting the immune system.

3 Creatine

Creatine supplementation enhances the body's ability to produce ATP, providing a rapid source of energy to fuel high-intensity activities such as weightlifting and sprinting. Consequently, it improves performance, supports muscular endurance, and increases muscle size and strength. Creatine is a vital supplement for competitive athletes or anyone seeking to optimize their resistance training or power-based sports performance.

4 Pre-Workout Formulas

Pre-workout supplements play a vital role in maximizing the effectiveness of training sessions by increasing energy, mental focus, physical endurance, and stamina. Ingredients like caffeine, nitric oxide precursors, and BCAAs prepare the body for intense workouts, reducing fatigue, and enhancing overall workout performance.

5 Fat Burners and Thermogenics

The importance of fat burners and thermogenic supplements lies in their ability to support weight-loss goals by enhancing metabolism, stimulating thermogenesis (the process of burning calories to produce heat), and moderating appetite. By optimizing the body's fat-burning potential, these supplements aid weight management when combined with a balanced diet and exercise program.

6 Vitamins and Minerals

Vitamins and minerals play essential roles in numerous metabolic and physiological processes throughout the body. They contribute to the proper functioning of the immune system, energy production, bone health, and overall well-being. Multivitamin and mineral supplements fill nutritional gaps in our diets and prevent potential deficiencies, ensuring that our bodies function optimally.

7 Omega-3 Fatty Acids

Omega-3 fatty acids play a crucial role in maintaining brain and cardiovascular health and reducing inflammation. They support cognitive function, memory, joint health, and mood regulation. Omega-3 supplements provide a concentrated source of these essential fatty acids, which are often lacking in our diets, especially for those who don't consume enough fatty fish or plant-based sources.

8 Probiotics and Digestive Enzymes

Probiotics and digestive enzymes play important roles in optimizing gut health, digestion, and the immune system. Probiotic supplements help restore the balance of beneficial bacteria in the gut, which is essential for nutrient absorption, immune function, and maintaining a healthy weight. Digestive enzymes facilitate the breakdown and absorption of various nutrients, ensuring our bodies can utilize the food we consume effectively.

9 Joint Support

Joint support supplements are essential for those experiencing joint pain, inflammation, and reduced mobility due to age, injury, or chronic conditions. They provide a combination of ingredients that promote joint health, maintain cartilage, and alleviate inflammation, significantly enhancing quality of life for those dealing with joint-related ailments.

10 Testosterone Boosters and Hormone Support

Testosterone boosters and hormone support supplements are critical for men seeking to achieve optimal hormonal balance, improve strength, and enhance sexual performance. These supplements can help combat the natural decline in testosterone levels associated with ageing or intense training, supporting overall vitality and well-being.

Chapter three

The Science Behind Fitness Supplements

3.1 Basics of Nutrition and Body Metabolism

To truly comprehend the underlying science that governs the efficacy of fitness supplements, it is imperative to possess a foundational understanding of nutrition and body metabolism. Grasping the basic concepts of how our bodies process nutrients and how these nutrients contribute to overall health and performance will enable consumers to make informed decisions about using fitness supplements to maximize their potential benefits. In this section, we delve into the basics of nutrition and body metabolism, providing invaluable insights into the science driving the fitness supplement industry.

1 Macronutrients

Macronutrients are the primary sources of energy and building blocks of our bodies, comprising carbohydrates, proteins, and fats.

- Carbohydrates

  Carbohydrates serve as the main energy source for the body and are broken down into glucose, fueling essential processes, including brain function and physical activity. Carbs can be classified as simple (e.g., sugars) or complex (e.g., starches and fibres), with complex carbohydrates being preferred due to their slower, more sustainable release of energy.

- Proteins

  Proteins are composed of amino acids, serving as the building blocks of our muscles, enzymes, hormones, and immune system components. Proteins help repair and build muscle tissue, maintain healthy skin and hair and facilitate numerous metabolic processes. Sources of protein include animal products, such as meat, fish, poultry, eggs, and dairy, as well as plant-based sources like beans, nuts, and seeds.

- Fats

Fats are a concentrated source of energy and are crucial for many physiological functions. They contribute to hormone production, cell membrane integrity, nutrient absorption, and insulation for our organs. Fats can be classified into saturated, monounsaturated, and polyunsaturated types, with the latter two (particularly omega-3 and omega-6 fatty acids) being essential for health.

2 Micronutrients

Micronutrients consist of vitamins and minerals, which are required in smaller quantities than macronutrients but are vital for maintaining optimal bodily function.

- Vitamins

  Vitamins are organic compounds that our bodies need for proper growth, development, repair, and maintenance. They are classified as either fat-soluble (vitamins A, D, E, K) or water-soluble (vitamin C, B-complex vitamins). Each vitamin has a specific role in the body, including supporting immune function, energy production, bone health, and antioxidant defence.

- Minerals

  Minerals are inorganic substances that have essential roles in the body, such as maintaining fluid balance, bone formation, and muscle function.

They can be classified as macro-minerals (calcium, phosphorus, magnesium, sodium, potassium, sulfur, and chlorine) or trace minerals (iron, zinc, copper, manganese, iodine, fluoride, and selenium), based on the amount required.

3 Body Metabolism

Metabolism encompasses all the chemical reactions and processes that occur within an organism to sustain life. The way our bodies convert food into energy and utilize the various nutrients for growth, repair, and physiological functions falls under metabolism.

- Basal Metabolic Rate (BMR)

  Basal metabolic rate (BMR) refers to the number of calories our bodies burn at rest to maintain basic physiological functions like respiration, circulation, and cell production. BMR is influenced by various factors, including age, sex, genetics, body composition, and hormone levels.

- Energy Expenditure

Energy expenditure comprises three components: basal metabolic rate (BMR), the thermic effect of food (TEF), and physical activity level (PAL). BMR accounts for about 60-70% of our total daily energy expenditure, with physical activity accounting for 15-30%, and TEF contributing about 10%.

- Metabolic Adaptation

Metabolic adaptation is the body's ability to adjust its energy expenditure in response to changes in energy intake and physical activity. These adaptations, such as increasing or decreasing metabolic rate, ensure that the body maintains energetic balance, preventing excessive weight gain or loss.

3.2 How Fitness Supplements Work

A comprehensive awareness of the science behind fitness supplements allows individuals to make educated decisions about which products to incorporate into their daily routines to achieve their health and fitness goals. Understanding the mechanisms through which these supplements exert their beneficial effects will enable consumers to select appropriate supplements that target specific needs and optimize their potential gains. In this section, we will explore how various fitness supplements work, shedding light on the complex interactions between these products and our bodies.

1 Protein Powders

Protein powders, such as whey, casein, or plant-based varieties, provide a concentrated and easily-absorbable source of amino acids needed for muscle-building and repair. They enhance muscle protein synthesis, prevent muscle breakdown, and speed up recovery following exercise. The positive nitrogen balance created by consuming protein powder plays a critical role in promoting anabolic (muscle-building) states and ensuring optimal muscle growth.

2 Amino Acids and BCAAs

Amino acids serve as the building blocks for proteins and are essential for various physiological functions, including enzyme activity. Branched-chain amino acids (BCAAs), comprising leucine, isoleucine, and valine, are particularly crucial for athletic performance. BCAAs stimulate muscle protein synthesis, reduce muscle soreness, and accelerate recovery. They also prevent muscle breakdown by inhibiting the activity of enzymes responsible for protein degradation, helping to preserve muscle mass during exercise.

3 Creatine

Creatine is a natural compound found in small amounts in certain foods and produced endogenously by the liver, kidneys, and pancreas. It plays a vital role in energy production by facilitating the conversion of adenosine diphosphate (ADP) back into adenosine triphosphate (ATP), our body's primary energy currency. Supplementation with creatine monohydrate increases intramuscular creatine stores, providing additional fuel for high-intensity activities, supporting muscle endurance, and promoting muscle size and strength gains.

4 Pre-Workout Formulas

Pre-workout supplements contain various ingredients that work synergistically to increase energy, boost mental focus, enhance physical endurance and stamina, and improve overall workout performance. Caffeine stimulates the central nervous system, increasing alertness and reducing perceived exertion. Nitric oxide precursors promote vasodilation, facilitating the delivery of oxygen and nutrients to working muscles.

5 Fat Burners and Thermogenics

Fat burners and thermogenic supplements support weight loss by increasing energy expenditure, stimulating metabolism, reducing appetite, and promoting the breakdown of stored fat. Ingredients like caffeine, green tea extract, and capsaicin work together to increase thermogenesis (the process of burning calories to produce heat), while other ingredients like L-carnitine support lipid transport and utilization.

6 Vitamins and Minerals

Vitamins and minerals are essential micronutrients our bodies require for proper functioning. Supplementation with multi-vitamins and minerals helps to fill nutritional gaps in our diets, ensuring we receive adequate levels of these essential nutrients. Vitamins play crucial roles in the immune system, energy production, bone health, and overall well-being, while minerals contribute to fluid balance, bone formation, and muscle function.

7 Omega-3 Fatty Acids

Omega-3 fatty acids, such as eicosapentaenoic acid (EPA) and docosahexaenoic acid (DHA), are essential polyunsaturated fats that support cognitive function, heart health, and inflammation modulation. Supplementation with omega-3 fatty acids helps to balance the ratio of omega-3 to omega-6 fatty acids in our bodies, which may become skewed with typical Western diets. This balance is critical in maintaining a healthy inflammatory response, preventing chronic disease, and supporting overall health.

8 Probiotics and Digestive Enzymes

Probiotic supplements contain live microorganisms that help restore the balance of beneficial bacteria in our gut microbiome, while digestive enzymes facilitate the breakdown and absorption of nutrients from the food we consume. Both probiotics and digestive enzymes help to optimize digestion, nutrient absorption, and gut health, leading to overall improvements in immune function, weight management, and general well-being.

9 Joint Support

Joint support supplements contain a combination of ingredients aimed at promoting joint health, maintaining cartilage, reducing inflammation, and providing a source of lubrication. Ingredients such as glucosamine, chondroitin, MSM, and hyaluronic acid work synergistically to ease joint discomfort, improve joint mobility, and support overall joint integrity.

10 Testosterone Boosters and Hormone Support

Testosterone boosters and hormone support supplements provide essential nutrients and natural ingredients like D-aspartic acid, ashwagandha, and fenugreek that help to regulate hormone balance, increase the synthesis of testosterone, and support overall male vitality. By optimizing hormonal balance, these supplements can contribute to improved mood, energy, libido, and muscle strength.

Chapter four

The Fitness Supplement Market

4.1 Overview of the Global Fitness Supplement Market

The global fitness supplement market has witnessed substantial growth over the last few years, driven by an increasing awareness of well-being, a rise in health consciousness, and a penchant for physical fitness. Technological advancements, innovative product formulations, and targeted marketing strategies have also played a significant role in shaping this thriving industry. In this section, we provide an in-depth analysis of the global fitness supplement market dynamics, exploring the key players, trends, and emerging opportunities within this lucrative business landscape.

1 Market Size and Growth

The fitness supplement market has been on an upward trajectory for years, with a steadily growing demand for high-quality, nutrient-dense products that cater to diverse consumer needs and preferences. According to recent market research data, the global fitness supplement market was valued at approximately USD 18.11 billion in 2021 and is projected to grow at a compound annual growth rate (CAGR) of 7.5% between 2022 and 2028, reaching an astonishing market valuation of over USD 30 billion by the end of this period. The burgeoning health and wellness industry, coupled with an increased emphasis on physical fitness, is largely responsible for driving this impressive growth.

2 Regional Analysis

Regionally, the global fitness supplement market is dominated by North America, primarily due to the robust presence of major industry players, a well-established fitness culture, and strong demand for supplements among fitness enthusiasts, athletes, and the general population. Europe occupies the second-largest market share, with a growing consumer base drawn to health and wellness trends, followed by the Asia-Pacific, Latin America, and Middle East & Africa regions.

The Asia-Pacific region, particularly countries like China, India, Japan, and South Korea, is poised for significant market growth in the coming years, driven by factors such as burgeoning middle-class populations, rapid urbanization, and an increased focus on maintaining a healthy lifestyle. The expansion of global supplement brands into these markets, coupled with strong local demand, creates a fertile ground for further market growth and investment opportunities.

3 Market Segmentation

The global fitness supplement market can be segmented based on product type, distribution channel, end-user demographics, and geographic region.

Product Type

The products can be categorized into protein powders, amino acids and BCAAs, creatine, pre-workout formulations, fat burners and thermogenics, vitamins and minerals, omega-3 fatty acids, probiotics and digestive enzymes, joint support, testosterone boosters and hormone support, among others. Protein powders and amino acids, particularly BCAAs, hold a substantial market share due to the crucial role of protein in muscle development, repair, and recovery, as well as emerging research on the benefits of amino acid supplementation.

Distribution Channel

Distribution channels for fitness supplements include e-commerce platforms, supermarkets and hypermarkets, drugstores and pharmacies, specialty stores, and others. E-commerce platforms continue to make significant gains in the market share, owing to the rapid growth of digital technology, the convenience of online shopping, and the abundant availability of product information and customer reviews.

End-User Demographics

Fitness supplements cater to a diverse range of consumers, including athletes and bodybuilders, recreational fitness enthusiasts, individuals seeking weight management solutions or general health maintenance, older adults requiring additional nutrients to address age-related concerns, and persons recovering from illness or surgery. Targeted marketing and innovative product offerings specifically tailored to each user group have contributed to the market expansion.

4 Key Market Players

Major players in the global fitness supplement market include:

- Glanbia plc
- Abbott Laboratories
- PepsiCo Inc.
- GNC Holdings Inc.
- Hormel Foods Corporation
- MusclePharm Corporation
- Clif Bar & Company
- Nutraceutical International Corporation
- Post Holdings, Inc.

The Nature's Bounty Co.

These key players account for a significant portion of the market share and maintain their competitive edge through strategic activities such as mergers and acquisitions, research and development, innovative product launches, and exploring potential growth areas.

5 Trends and Opportunities

Several notable trends and opportunities are shaping the global fitness supplement market landscape:

1. Personalized and customized supplements cater to individual needs and preferences, utilizing AI-generated nutritional recommendations based on factors such as genetics, lifestyle, and fitness goals.

2. Plant-based, vegan, and organic supplements are in high demand due to consumers' growing

concerns surrounding environmental sustainability and ethical consumption.

3. Emerging research on novel ingredients and their potential benefits promises the development of innovative and groundbreaking fitness supplement products.

4. Collaborations with professional athletes, influencers, and celebrities continue to expand brand reach and awareness through endorsement and marketing efforts.

4.2 Notable Trends and Key Players

The global fitness supplement market is a sophisticated, dynamic landscape, shaped by various forces that continuously redefine and reinvent the industry. The trends we see today are influenced by several factors, including shifting consumer preferences, technological advancements, and research breakthroughs. Here, we delve into the notable trends shaping the fitness supplement market and discuss key players that have a substantial impact on its progression.

1 Notable Trends in the Fitness Supplement Market

1. Personalization of Fitness Supplements

    One of the most notable trends revolves around the customization and personalization of fitness supplements. Companies have begun tailoring their products to meet individual dietary needs and fitness goals. From products designed specifically for women and men to formulations that account for age, dietary restrictions, and health conditions, these tailored solutions have become a rising trend.

2. Natural and Plant-Based Supplements

    A growing interest in natural and plant-based products is shaping the fitness supplement market.

Consumers are gradually moving away from artificial and synthetic ingredients, gravitating towards plant-derived proteins, vitamins, and antioxidants. This rise in demand is driven by a broader societal trend for sustainable and environmentally-friendly products.

3. Clean Label Products

The desire for transparency has spurred the advent of clean-label products. Consumers want to know precisely what goes into their supplements, and they're demanding simplicity and clarity. This trend has led manufacturers to reduce their ingredients lists, eliminate artificial additives and preservatives, and use clear, easy-to-understand labels.

4. Functional Foods

Functional foods, or foods that have a positive effect on health beyond basic nutrition, are growing in popularity in the fitness supplement market.

These include enriched protein bars, dairy products infused with probiotics, or drinks enhanced with vitamins and minerals. The convenience and multifunctionality of these products make them very appealing to health-conscious consumers leading busy lifestyles.

5. Technological Innovation

   Technology is also shaping the industry. From apps that recommend supplement regimes based on personal health data to AI and machine learning algorithms used to predict consumer behaviour and optimize product development, the supplement industry is becoming more tech-focused.

2 Key Players in the Fitness Supplement Market

1. Glanbia plc

Irish-based Glanbia plc has been a significant player in the fitness supplement market. Renowned for popular brands like Optimum Nutrition, BSN, and Isopure, Glanbia's product portfolio is impressive and diversified, covering an array of fitness and nutritional needs.

2. Abbott Laboratories

Abbott Laboratories, a multinational medical devices and healthcare company, provides a range of supplements to promote various health aspects. Their products, including Ensure, Glucerna, and Similac, form a substantial part of the nutrition and fitness supplement market.

3. PepsiCo Inc.

PepsiCo, recently extended its portfolio to fitness nutrition with the acquisitions of MTY Food Group and Muscle Milk producer CytoSport Holdings, bolstering their presence in the fitness supplement market.

4. MusclePharm Corporation

MusclePharm is an award-winning company renowned for its safe, effective, and scientifically backed fitness supplements. Its product line includes proteins, pre-workouts, BCAAs, amino acids, and more.

5. The Nature's Bounty Co.

The Nature's Bounty Co., known for its vitamins and dietary supplements, has brands like Solgar, Sundown, MET-Rx, and Pure Protein under its umbrella, making it a key player in the fitness supplement market.

Chapter Five

Consumer Behavior and Fitness Supplements

5.1 Factors Influencing Purchase Decisions

In an industry as dynamic as that of fitness supplements, it is crucial to understand the factors influencing consumer behaviour and purchase decisions. In this age of information and increased health consciousness, customers are becoming exceedingly discerning, particularly when it comes to health products. In this section, we will explore the key determinants that influence consumer behaviour in the fitness supplement market.

1 Quality of the Product

The perceived quality of fitness supplements significantly influences consumer purchase behaviour. Consumers are particularly responsive to the quality of ingredients, formulation, purity, safety, and efficacy of the product. Products that can demonstrate scientific backing, proven efficacy, and superior quality are likely to be more appealing to consumers.

2 Price

Price remains a pivotal factor influencing consumer behaviour in the fitness supplement market. However, the price sensitivity varies across different consumer segments. Some consumers may be willing to pay a premium for high-quality, clinically proven, or organic products. In contrast, others may be looking for the most cost-effective option that provides necessary benefits.

3 Brand Reputation

Brand reputation has a significant influence on consumer purchase decisions. Brands that have a solid track record, positive customer reviews, and are known for their adherence to quality and safety standards are more likely to attract customers. The brand image gets tied up with factors such as trust, reliability, and consumers' perceptions of the brand's values.

4 Personal Health Goals

A consumer's personal health and fitness goals significantly impact their selection of fitness supplements. For instance, athletes or fitness enthusiasts might prefer supplements that focus on muscle growth, recovery, or performance. Simultaneously, individuals with weight management or general wellness goals might prefer products designed for those purposes.

5 Product Accessibility

Consumers are likely to favour brands and products that are easily accessible. This factor includes both, physical availability in local or online stores, and the ease of understanding the product (clear labelling, detailed product information). As online shopping continues to surge, brands with a strong e-commerce presence are likely to have a distinct advantage.

6 Social Influence

The influence of social circles, including friends, family, fitness trainers, and even social media influencers, play a significant role in consumer purchase decisions. Recommendations from trusted sources or endorsements from admired figures can significantly impact a consumer's choice of fitness supplements.

7 Advertising and Marketing Efforts

Effective advertising and marketing strategies can significantly steer consumer purchase behaviour. From striking packaging to compelling advertisements, well-planned marketing tactics can create brand awareness, spark interest, and ultimately, drive sales.

5.2 Marketing Strategies in the Supplement Industry

In the highly competitive supplement industry, effective marketing strategies are key to gaining an edge in the marketplace. From raising brand awareness and attracting new customers, to building loyalty and boosting sales, marketing strategies work on multiple fronts to drive business growth. In this section, we will examine some compelling marketing strategies used in the supplement industry to effectively align with consumer behavior and preferences.

1 Product Differentiation

Owing to the crowded supplement market, product differentiation is a cornerstone marketing strategy. In a bid for uniqueness, companies are focusing on creating groundbreaking formulations, specialized supplements, and products catering to specific demographic groups and health concerns. Natural, organic, vegan, non-GMO, gluten-free, sugar-free – all serve to differentiate a product and target specific consumer groups.

2 Influencer Marketing

In the current digital age, influencer marketing is becoming growlingly influential. Brands are collaborating with fitness trainers, athletes, health bloggers, celebrities, and other influencers, leveraging their popularity to reach a broader audience. As consumers often trust recommendations from personalities they admire, this can be an effective way to boost product visibility and credibility.

3 Social Media and Content Marketing

Utilizing social media platforms and deploying compelling content marketing strategies allow businesses to reach and engage their target audience. Sharing valuable content, from product insights, health tips, fitness routines, customer testimonials, to interactive posts can help brands establish a strong online presence, engage customers and build brand loyalty.

4 Educational Marketing

Since supplements tie into people's health and well-being, providing detailed, transparent and educational content can build consumer trust. This could include blog articles, webinars, ebooks, infographics, or explainer videos around nutrition, supplement effectiveness, their pros and cons, usage instructions, and impact.

5 Personalization

Understanding the specific needs and preferences of customers allows for personalized marketing efforts. Today, with access to a wealth of consumer data and advanced technological tools, brands can offer personalized product recommendations, tailored content, promotional offers, and customer experiences.

6 Free Samples and Trials

Free samples and trials offer consumers a risk-free way to try products before buying, thereby lowering the barrier to purchasing. Supplement brands can offer these at gyms, health clubs, wellness events or as part of online promotions.

7 Partnership and Collaborations

Partnering with fitness centres, wellness clinics, sports clubs, dieticians, and even restaurants and cafes can help supplement businesses to expand their reach. Such collaborations may involve product placements, combined offerings, joint promotions, or endorsement deals.

Chapter six

Creating a Fitness Supplement

6.1 Steps in Developing a New Supplement

Developing a new fitness supplement encompasses numerous steps and facets, from initial concept and formulation to production and marketing. In this section, we will detail the systematic process involved in bringing a new fitness supplement to market.

1 Market Research

The entire process begins with robust market research. Understanding current trends, consumer needs, competitor products, regulatory requirements, and potential gaps in the market is crucial. This phase involves analyzing your target consumers' likes, dislikes, preferences, and demands.

2 Concept Development

Based on market research, generate product concepts that can potentially fulfill market needs. This could include a unique combination of ingredients, catering to a specific dietary trend, or serving a particular demographic. Concept development should also consider brand alignment, pricing strategies, and feasibility.

3 Formulation

This is the scientific step where biochemists and nutritionists determine the specific blend of ingredients to be included in the supplement. The formulation should be based on scientific research and must comply with dietary supplement regulations. Additionally, a balance must be achieved between the effectiveness of the formulation and its taste and texture.

4 Prototyping and Testing

Once the formulation is finalized, a prototype or sample batch of the supplement is produced. This is followed by in-depth testing to ensure quality, safety, effectiveness, and consumer acceptability. Testing involves laboratory analysis and possibly consumer trials, all while complying with safety protocols and regulations.

5 Manufacturing Process

Post approval from testing, the manufacturing process begins. This phase often involves collaboration with a certified supplement manufacturer to ensure high production standards. Key considerations at this stage include ingredient sourcing, production costs, quality assurance, packaging, and meeting regulatory compliances.

6 Branding and Packaging

Branding and packaging are vital aspects of product development. Packaging and label design should reflect the brand image, attract the target audience, and clearly display the necessary information about the product. Additionally, the supplement's name, logo, taglines, and overall branding should resonate with consumers and the market niche.

7 Marketing and Promotion

A comprehensive marketing strategy is developed and executed to promote the new supplement. This may include social media marketing, influencer collaborations, content marketing, SEO, PR campaigns, trade shows, sales promotions, and more.

8 Sales and Distribution

Establishing efficient sales and distribution channels is the final step. This involves partnering with fitness studios, supplement stores, pharmacies, or online e-commerce platforms, to ensure the product reaches the intended target audience.

6.2 Importance of Quality Control and Testing

Fitness supplements directly impact consumers' health and wellbeing. Consequently, ensuring high-quality standards, product safety, and effectiveness is paramount. Quality control and rigorous testing are integral aspects of supplement development, setting the foundation for consumer trust and loyalty. In this section, we will explore the importance and key benefits of quality control and testing protocols in the fitness supplement industry.

1 Ensuring Safety and Compliance with Regulations

One of the primary functions of quality control and testing is ensuring the safety of the supplement for consumer use. Identifying and eliminating potential impurities, toxins, or harmful substances during the production process is critical. Additionally, quality control measures ensure that the supplement manufacturing process complies with FDA guidelines and Good Manufacturing Practices (GMP).

2 Confirming Product Efficacy

Quality control testing encompasses evaluating the formulation's effectiveness and the product's overall efficacy. Establishing the optimal dosage, bioavailability, and potency of the supplement is vital for achieving desired results. Testing protocols should verify that the product delivers the intended benefits and is clinically-proven.

.3 Standardizing Consistency

Consistency is an essential factor in customer satisfaction and brand loyalty. Rigorous quality control ensures that each batch of the supplement adheres to the established formula and is consistent in taste, texture, and performance. Maintaining uniformity across batches ensures that customers receive a consistent experience with every purchase.

4 Reinforcing Customer Trust and Brand Reputation

Consumer trust is the bedrock upon which successful supplement brands are built. By ensuring high-quality standards and robust testing processes, brands can demonstrate their commitment to customer welfare and satisfaction, earning trust over time. A solid reputation bolstered by quality and safety fosters long-term customer loyalty and can command higher price points and market prominence.

5 Reducing Risks and Liability

Implementing strict quality control processes helps reduce the risks associated with product recalls or negative consumer experiences. Proactively addressing quality issues before products reach the market minimizes the potential for liability issues and protects the brand from reputational damage.

6 Supporting Marketing Claims

In a market driven by consumer expectations, marketing claims can play a significant role in purchase decisions. Demonstrating that a supplement has undergone thorough quality control testing and adheres to stringent safety standards strengthens the credibility of marketing claims and creates a sense of reliability.

Chapter Seven
Branding and Packaging

7.1 Importance of Branding in the Supplement Industry

In the saturated field of the fitness supplements industry, strong and effective branding is a potent tool for differentiation, consumer connection, and business growth. Branding, coupled with impactful packaging, creates a first impression and sets the tone for the consumer's entire experience with a supplement product. This section will dissect the critical role that branding and packaging play in the success of fitness supplements.

1 Creation of a Unique Identity

At the heart of effective branding is the formation of a unique identity. A strong brand identity includes everything from the visual elements like the logo and colour scheme to the brand values and tone of communication. This identity becomes synonymous with the product and helps differentiate it from competitors in the crowded supplement market.

2 Telling the Brand Story

Branding allows a company to tell its story. The brand's history, mission, vision, and values can all be communicated through strategic branding. A compelling brand story can foster an emotional connection with consumers, which extends beyond the product's functional benefits.

3 Building Trust and Credibility

Branding helps foster trust and credibility with consumers. Brands that consistently deliver on their promises and maintain high standards of quality and service become trusted by consumers. This trust can lead to long-term customer loyalty, repeat purchases, and positive word-of-mouth recommendations.

4 Influencing Purchase Decisions

Branding and packaging play a significant role in influencing consumer purchasing decisions. Attractive, clear, and informative packaging can not only catch consumers' eyes on retail shelves or online listings but can also provide critical information about the supplement that influences buying decisions.

5 Enhancing Visibility and Recognition

Well-executed branding makes a product easily identifiable and memorable. The colours, logo, and design elements used in branding and packaging contribute to creating a visual image in consumers' minds. Over time, this recognition can improve the brand's visibility and reputation in the market.

6 Communicating Product Quality and Value

Effective branding and packaging can communicate the quality and value of the supplement. High-quality design elements, professional and appealing packaging, and clear communication of product benefits and features can convey the product's superiority and justify a premium price point.

7.2 Innovations in Packaging and Designing

With the expanding dietary supplement market, innovative packaging and design have become increasingly critical in creating a successful product. Innovation aids in adapting to changing consumer preferences, environmental challenges, and standing out in the crowded supplement market. In this section, we delve into several recent innovations in the realms of packaging and design that are shaping the fitness supplements industry.

1 Sustainable Packaging

As environmental awareness grows among consumers, brands are responding by incorporating sustainable practices in their packaging. This includes using biodegradable or recyclable materials, reducing unnecessary packaging, and utilizing post-consumer waste. Sustainable packaging not only lessens environmental impact but also appeals to environmentally conscious consumers, creating a win-win situation for both the brand and the planet.

2 Interactive Packaging

Technology has paved the way for interactive packaging, where QR codes, augmented reality, or NFC technologies are used to provide consumers with additional product information, usage guidelines, or even immersive brand experiences. This form of packaging is more engaging and boosts the customer experience by providing value beyond the product itself.

3 Flexible and Portable Packaging

The rise of on-the-go lifestyles has prompted innovations in convenient and portable supplement packaging. Single-serving sachets, stick packs, and resealable pouches cater to consumers seeking practicality. They offer a "grab-and-go" convenience, ensuring that regular supplement intake isn't disrupted by a busy schedule or travel.

4 Child-Resistant Packaging

Safety is paramount in the supplement industry, and one significant innovation in this field is child-resistant packaging. These designs, including push-and-turn caps or perforated breakables, restrict children's access while still being user-friendly for adults, thereby minimizing unintentional ingestion by young children.

5 Transparent Packaging

In an era where consumers value transparency, clear packaging designs are gaining popularity. Whether literal, with see-through materials, or figurative, with detailed product labels, transparency in packaging helps establish trust and allows consumers to know exactly what they are purchasing.

6 Personalization

With the rise of personalised health and wellness, brands are adopting packaging designs that reflect an individual's needs or preferences. This can range from customised supplement blends with personalised labels to flexible subscription models where packaging is tailored to the frequency of use.

Chapter eight

Marketing and Selling Fitness Supplements

8.1 Effective Marketing Strategies

The fitness supplement market is dynamic and highly competitive, with numerous offerings vying for consumer attention. Breaking through the noise requires strategic and compelling marketing tactics. This section will explore effective marketing strategies that fitness supplement brands can deploy to capture market share and boost sales.

1 Identify and Understand Your Target Audience

Every effective marketing strategy starts with understanding the target audience. By identifying who the ideal consumers are (their age, gender, fitness goals, lifestyle, preferences, etc.), brands can tailor their product development, messaging, and marketing to cater to their specific needs, wants, and expectations.

2 Highlight Unique Selling Proposition (USP)

Every brand must identify its unique selling proposition (USP) and work to communicate it effectively. Whether it's a unique ingredient, superior formulation, third-party certifications, or an innovative delivery system, highlighting these distinguishing factors can help a fitness supplement stand out from the crowd.

3 Utilize Content Marketing

Content marketing, including blog posts, videos, infographics, and e-books, can provide value to consumers and establish the brand as a reliable resource within the fitness supplements industry. Educational and engaging content can also improve search engine visibility, driving organic traffic and potential sales.

4 Invest in Influencer Marketing

With the rise of social media and fitness influencers, leveraging influencer partnerships can be a highly effective strategy. Endorsements from trusted fitness experts and influencers can improve brand visibility, create a buzz, and drive sales.

5 Leverage Social Media Platforms

Social media platforms are invaluable tools for marketing fitness supplements. Brands can use these platforms to engage with consumers, share impactful content, run advertising campaigns, and gather consumer feedback. A well-strategized and executed social media plan can significantly improve brand visibility and consumer engagement.

6 Utilize Email Marketing

Email marketing can be an excellent strategy for retaining existing customers and encouraging repeat purchases. By offering valuable content, exclusive deals, and personalized recommendations via email, brands can nurture relationships with their customers and boost their lifetime value.

7 Highlight Testimonials and Reviews

Sharing positive customer testimonials and reviews on website, social media, and other marketing collateral can significantly influence buying decisions. These reviews can add to the sense of credibility and trustworthiness often needed in the supplement industry.

Chapter nine

Legal and Regulatory Considerations

9.1 Regulations Governing the Fitness Supplement Industry

Navigating the legal and regulatory landscape is essential in the fitness supplement industry. Country-specific laws and regulations can vary, but in general, robust systems are in place to ensure the safety, efficacy, and accurate representation of products. This section will discuss some key regulations governing the fitness supplement industry to help businesses sail smoothly in the sea of legal and regulatory requirements.

1 Dietary Supplement Definition and Classification

The first step in regulatory compliance is understanding the definition and classification of dietary supplements. In the United States, supplements are classified as a subcategory of food, governed by the Food and Drug Administration (FDA) and the Federal Trade Commission (FTC). The European Food Safety Authority (EFSA) regulates supplements in the European Union, where they are classified as food supplements.

2 Ingredient and Safety Regulations

One of the cornerstones of regulation in the fitness supplement industry is the safety and efficacy of ingredients. Depending on the country or region, certain ingredients may be prohibited, restricted, or require specific precautionary measures. In the US, the FDA requires manufacturers to ensure the safety of ingredients under the Dietary Supplement Health and Education Act of

1994 (DSHEA). In Europe, the EFSA evaluates and places restrictions on some ingredients and sets maximum allowable levels for vitamins and minerals.

3 Good Manufacturing Practices (GMP)

To ensure the quality of fitness supplements, manufacturers must adhere to good manufacturing practices (GMP). These practices encompass all aspects of the production process, from ingredient sourcing to labelling and packaging. Compliance with GMP regulations, such as the Code of Federal Regulations Title 21 (21 CFR) in the US, helps ensure product quality and reduce the risk of contamination or mislabeling.

4 Labeling Regulations

Accurate and informative labelling is another crucial aspect of regulatory compliance in the fitness supplement industry. Labels must accurately list all ingredients, allergen information, recommended serving sizes, health warnings, and other essential information. In the US, the FDA issues specific labelling requirements under the DSHEA, while in the EU, products must adhere to the Food Information for Consumers Regulation (EU) No. 1169/2011.

5 Health Claims and Advertising

Health claims made by fitness supplement brands—on the product label, in advertisements, or through other marketing channels—must comply with specific regulations to avoid misleading consumers. In the US, the FDA and FTC regulate health claims, requiring them to be supported by scientific evidence. In the EU, the EFSA approves specific health claims to ensure that they are accurate and rooted in scientific proof.

6 Product Registration and Notifications

In some countries or regions, new dietary supplement products might require registration with or notification to relevant authorities. For example, in Europe, companies must notify relevant competent authorities before placing a new food supplement on the market.

9.2 Dealing with Legal Challenges

Legal challenges in the fitness supplement industry can range from regulatory non-compliance to intellectual property disputes and product liability issues. Businesses must actively address these challenges to maintain their reputation, protect consumer safety, and minimize the risk of legal repercussions. This section will provide guidance on dealing with legal challenges in the fitness supplement industry.

1 Establish and Maintain Regulatory Compliance

Proactively establishing and maintaining regulatory compliance is essential for businesses operating in the fitness supplement industry. Familiarize yourself with relevant regulations that apply to your products, such as ingredient restrictions, GMPs, labelling requirements, and health claims. Regularly monitor any updates or changes to these regulations to ensure ongoing compliance.

2 Intellectual Property Protection

Intellectual property (IP) protection is crucial for fitness supplement companies with unique formulations, brand names, packaging designs, or marketing strategies. Registering trademarks, copyrights, and patents can help protect your brand equity, safeguard your innovations, and reduce the likelihood of legal disputes.

3 Legal Expertise and Resources

Hiring legal counsel with expertise in the fitness supplement industry can be invaluable in dealing with legal challenges. Skilled attorneys can help identify potential issues, provide guidance on maintaining compliance, and represent businesses in legal disputes. Additionally, they can aid in negotiating licensing agreements, contracts, and various other legal documents.

4 Establish a Compliance Management System

Implement a comprehensive compliance management system to monitor all aspects of regulatory compliance, from ingredient sourcing to product labelling and claims. Allocate roles and responsibilities within your organization, ensure clear communication and reporting, and regularly update your practices according to regulatory changes and industry best practices.

5 Maintain Transparency and Communication

Clear communication and transparency is essential in managing legal challenges. Be proactive in communicating relevant information to consumers, suppliers, and regulators. Establish a system for addressing consumer inquiries and concerns. Developing trust with stakeholders by being open and honest about your products and practices can help mitigate potential legal issues.

6 Be Prepared for Product Recalls

In the unfortunate event of a product recall, having a well-prepared plan is crucial. Develop a product recall procedure that includes steps for identifying the affected products, communicating with suppliers, distributors, consumers, and regulatory authorities, as well as measures to remedy the situation. Swift action in the face of a recall can help protect consumer safety and minimize legal and reputational risks.

7 Carry Appropriate Insurance Coverage

Carrying the appropriate business insurance coverage, such as product liability insurance, can help mitigate financial losses resulting from legal disputes or claims related to your fitness supplements. Consult with an insurance professional to assess your specific needs and obtain suitable coverage.

Conclusion

The business of creating and selling fitness supplements is a complex yet rewarding endeavour that not only offers a lucrative opportunity but also impacts people's health and wellness. From understanding market dynamics and consumer demand, product development and manufacturing, to marketing strategies and regulatory compliance, each aspect plays a critical role in ensuring business success.

Understanding customer needs is at the heart of a successful fitness supplement business. With a diverse target audience ranging from professional athletes to health-conscious individuals, creating the right product that caters to their specific needs is paramount. Deciphering this complex interplay of demographics, psychographics, behavior, needs, wants, and expectations plays an integral role in developing an effective product line-up.

Product development and manufacturing is a core area where success is hinged on combining scientific research, quality ingredients, and best manufacturing practices. Sound knowledge of nutrition science and industry trends is crucial to ideate, innovate, and deliver safe, effective, and differentiated products that resonate with consumers and build brand loyalty.

Marketing contributes immensely to the growth and profitability of the fitness supplement enterprise. With strategies ranging from identifying and showcasing USPs, leveraging social media, partnering with influencers, providing educational content, and valuing consumer testimonials, businesses can enhance their brand visibility and drive sales.

On the other hand, the fitness supplement industry is bound by several laws and regulations intended to protect consumer safety and ensure fair trade. Businesses must navigate the regulatory landscape diligently to comply with ingredient safety, manufacturing practices, labeling, and health claims. Understanding these nuances helps brands prevent potential legal challenges and maintain a trustworthy, respectful relationship with consumers and regulatory bodies.